ALZHEIMER'S ROADMAP:

Advance Directives, Durable Power of Attorney, Wills, and Other Legal Considerations

Laura Town and Karen Kassel

Silver Hills Press
Zionsville, IN 46077

ISBN: 978-1-943414-00-0

Production Credits:
Authors: Laura Town and Karen Kassel
Publisher: Silver Hills Press
Photos: All images used under license from Shutterstock.com

Social Media Connections:
Laura Town
Twitter: @laurawtown
LinkedIn: https://www.linkedin.com/in/lauratown
GooglePlus: https://plus.google.com/u/0/117415714202281042310/posts
Pinterest: https://www.pinterest.com/laurat0428

Karen Kassel
Twitter: @KarenKassel1
LinkedIn: www.linkedin.com/pub/karen-kassel/62/2b/915/

TABLE OF CONTENTS

ADVANCE DIRECTIVES, DURABLE POWER OF ATTORNEY, WILLS, AND OTHER LEGAL CONSIDERATIONS 1

    Checklist: Legal documents needed for individuals with Alzheimer's disease 2

Elder Law Attorneys..**2**

    Checklist: How to find a good elder law attorney....................................... 3

    Checklist: How to prepare for your elder law attorney appointment.................... 5

    Checklist: Topics to discuss with your elder law attorney 7

    Checklist: Reasons to review legal documents.. 7

Discussing Legal Documents **9**

    Checklist: How to discuss legal documents with your loved one.......................... 10

Legal Documents for Healthcare..**12**

Durable Power of Attorney for Healthcare **12**

    Checklist: Basics about a durable power of attorney for healthcare 13

    Checklist: Responsibilities of the principal.. 14

    Checklist: Characteristics of a good healthcare agent............................. 15

    Checklist: Responsibilities of a healthcare agent...................................... 16

Advance Directives **19**

Living Will...**20**

    Checklist: Basics about a living will... 20

    Checklist: Medical treatments that may be covered in a living will..................... 21

    Checklist: Responsibilities of the principal.. 22

    Checklist: Situations to consider when deciding about life-prolonging medical procedures.. 22

Do Not Resuscitate (DNR) and Do Not Intubate (DNI) Orders.............**23**

    Checklist: Basics about DNR and DNI orders 24

    Checklist: When should my loved one have a DNR order?.................................. 25

    Checklist: When should my loved one NOT have a DNR order?...................... 26

Artificial Nutrition and Hydration **27**

    Checklist: Basics about artificial nutrition and hydration 27

Organ, Tissue, and Body Donation 28

Checklist: Basics about organ, tissue, and body donation 28

Other Medical Directives 29

Checklist: Basics about less-common medical directives.......................29

Physician Orders for Life-Sustaining Treatment (POLST) 31

Legal Documents for Finances 31

Durable Power of Attorney for Finances 32

Checklist: Basics about a durable power of attorney for finances.......32

Checklist: Responsibilities of the principal...33

Checklist: Characteristics of a good attorney-in-fact...........................33

Checklist: Responsibilities of an attorney-in-fact................................34

Last Will and Testament...36

Checklist: Basics about a last will and testament.................................36

Checklist: Responsibilities of the testator...38

Checklist: Items commonly listed in the will 39

Checklist: Characteristics of a good executor of the will 42

Checklist: Responsibilities of an executor of the will 42

Trusts 43

Checklist: Terms related to trusts 43

Checklist: Types of trusts..44

Checklist: What to put in a trust 45

Checklist: How do I know if my loved one needs a trust?...................45

Checklist: How do I help my loved one create a trust?........................46

Checklist: Characteristics of a good trustee 47

Checklist: Responsibilities of a trustee..48

Other Legal Documents and Roles...48

Power of Attorney 49

General Power of Attorney 49

Springing Power of Attorney 49

Healthcare Proxy 50

Conservator and/or Guardian 50

Guardian of Minor Children **51**

Checklist: Things to consider when choosing a good guardian for children 52

Administrator **53**

Representative Payee and/or VA Fiduciary **53**

Social Media Will **53**

Ethical Will **54**

Dealing with Conflict **54**

Checklist: Common causes of conflict 55

Checklist: Strategies to prevent or resolve conflict 56

Conclusion **58**

ABOUT THE AUTHORS **59**

A NOTE FROM THE AUTHORS **61**

RESOURCES **63**

REFERENCE LIST **67**

ADVANCE DIRECTIVES, DURABLE POWER OF ATTORNEY, WILLS, AND OTHER LEGAL CONSIDERATIONS

A diagnosis of Alzheimer's disease can be devastating to you and your loved one. All individuals with Alzheimer's disease eventually become unable to make good decisions about their healthcare and finances. Therefore, having written legal documents in place that help you know your loved one's wishes will relieve some of the burden of making hard choices about medical care and help avoid conflict between family members over possessions and healthcare decisions.

With my (Laura) dad's disease journey, we endured a lot of drama. He got lost in France, he was convinced that Nigerians were going to kidnap him, and he hitchhiked. I was fortunate, however, that he was docile and agreeable when I decided to take control over his financial and legal affairs. I think he was at the point where he knew he needed that. One of my childhood friends, Amy, had a completely different experience. Her dad refused to allow Amy to even know where the checkbook was, much less sign off on any legal or financial papers that would give her any control.

As in Amy's case, your loved one may resent you for asking them to turn over legal control of their finances or healthcare to you or another trusted individual. This resentment is part of the disease process, and it is something you will have to make peace with. Unfortunately, nothing is easy about helping a loved one endure Alzheimer's disease. You can only do the best you can for your loved one and accept the hurt feelings that result, knowing that your loved one's responses are caused by the disease and their fear of losing independence.

Because your loved one must be legally competent to sign legal documents pertaining to healthcare and finances, you should help them prepare these documents as soon as possible. The checklist below provides a list of legal documents your loved one should prepare now before they are no longer able to share their wishes with you. These documents will ensure that your loved one's wishes are being met even if they can no longer make their preferences known. This book will describe these and other documents, what you need to prepare each document, and the responsibilities of individuals named in the documents.

Checklist: Legal documents needed for individuals with Alzheimer's disease

Recommended:

☐ Durable Power of Attorney for Healthcare

☐ Durable Power of Attorney for Finances

☐ Living Will

☐ Last Will and Testament

Optional:

☐ Living Trust

☐ Do Not Resuscitate (DNR)

Elder Law Attorneys

Legal documents can be confusing, and different states have different requirements and different terminology for legal documents pertaining to healthcare and finances. Therefore, searching for a trusted elder law attorney is a good starting point for many families with a loved one who was recently diagnosed with Alzheimer's disease.

Elder law attorneys specialize in legal documents related to elderly care, including options for healthcare, distributing possessions, and receiving Medicare or Medicaid services. Elder law attorneys will understand your state's requirements for documents such as living wills and Do Not Resuscitate (DNR) orders. They will also know the proper procedures for appointing a power of attorney for your loved one.

If your loved one does not already have legal documents in place, you should find a good elder law attorney as quickly as possible after your loved one's diagnosis, because it is important for your loved one to be able to make decisions about legal matters while they can still understand and give consent to the documents. (This is

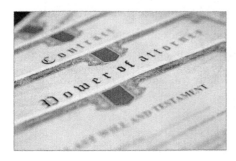

called "legal capacity" or "competency.") Once your loved one's mental abilities begin to decline, they are no longer qualified to sign legal documents, and it will be easier for family members to contest the documents if they don't agree with the stipulations in those documents.

I'll admit it, I'm cheap. In my dad's case, I was hoping that I could prepare legal documents on the Internet or with the use of legal software. However, when I met with the elder law attorney we chose, she brought up scenarios that I had not contemplated. She also told us ways we could effectively protect Dad's assets and handle the taxes that I would not have known about. Even though I spent $250 per hour for the attorney, I was relieved. The legal advice I received saved me more in the long run than if I had relied on software that could not possibly take into account my particular circumstances.

Having a good elder law attorney can help ease some stress, but how should you go about finding the right attorney for your needs? The following checklist provides some good questions to ask when searching for an elder law attorney.

Checklist: How to find a good elder law attorney

☐ Does this attorney live in my area? You can find attorneys in your area by searching online or in the phone book for elder law attorneys. There is also a national registry for elder law attorneys at http://www.naela.org/.

☐ Does this attorney understand my state's requirements for legal documents?

☐ Does this attorney handle all the legal documents I need to make? For example, do they understand estate law, trust law, healthcare decision making, and senior housing options?

☐ Does this attorney understand Medicare and Medicaid requirements, and will they be able to make suggestions and handle paperwork regarding qualifications for Medicare and Medicaid?

☐ How long has this attorney been practicing elder law?

☐ What percentage of this attorney's practice focuses on elder law?

☐ Is this attorney a Certified Elder Law Attorney?

☐ Is this attorney active in any professional and community organizations?

☐ Is there a fee for the first consultation? If so, what is it?

☐ How does this attorney charge fees? By the hour? By the document? What is the hourly or per document rate? Can my loved one afford these fees?

☐ How frequently does this attorney bill my loved one? Weekly? Monthly? Upon completion of work?

☐ Does this attorney charge for out-of-pocket expenses like copies, postage, etc.?

☐ Does this attorney charge for over-the-phone consultations or questions?

☐ Will this attorney require a retainer? (A retainer is money paid to the attorney before work starts, and the attorney pays himself or herself from these funds.)

☐ How long is a typical wait period for getting an appointment with this attorney?

☐ Is this attorney able to handle decision-making responsibilities in my absence?

☐ Is this attorney willing to be an executor or administrator of my loved one's estate if I need this service?

☐ Will this attorney provide advice on how to "spend down" my loved one's assets to help qualify for Medicaid, if I decide to do this? (See *Long-Term Care Insurance, Power of Attorney, Wealth Management, and Other First Steps* for Medicaid qualification requirements.)

☐ Is this attorney willing to be a mediator between family members in the event of family disagreements?

☐ Is this attorney familiar with local long-term care facilities and the practices they follow in accepting or denying patients?

☐ How frequently does this attorney recommend reviewing legal documents to make sure they are up to date? What is the fee for this service?

☐ Do I know anyone who has used this attorney? If so, do they recommend this attorney?

☐ Are there any online reviews about this attorney or law firm? If so, are they generally positive or negative reviews?

Once you or your loved one has contacted several elder law attorneys and selected the one that is the best fit for your loved one's needs, how should you prepare for that first appointment? The checklist below details the information you will need to gather before your first appointment with an elder law attorney.

Checklist: How to prepare for your elder law attorney appointment

- ☐ Gather information about your loved one's personal records, including legal name; Social Security number; place and date of birth; locations of legal documents such as birth certificates and marriage certificates; and education, employment, and military records.

- ☐ Gather information about your loved one's medical condition, including diagnosis, current stage of illness, and ability to care for themselves.

- ☐ Determine the overall financial needs and resources of your loved one. Will your loved one have enough in savings and retirement income to cover their needs? Will your loved one qualify for federal or state financial assistance?

- ☐ Gather documents related to your loved one's bank accounts, including checking accounts, savings accounts, and certificates of deposit.

- ☐ Gather documents related to your loved one's recent federal and state tax returns.

- ☐ Gather documents related to your loved one's sources of income, such as Social Security, disability, pensions, retirement accounts, veterans benefits, investments, rental property, and other income.

- ☐ Gather documents related to your loved one's investments, including stocks, bonds, mutual funds, and other investments.

- ☐ Gather documents related to your loved one's property, including real estate, vehicles, and personal possessions, especially valuable possessions such as jewelry. Also determine whether your loved one has a safe deposit box and what the box contains.

- ☐ Gather documents related to your loved one's insurance policies, including health insurance, home insurance, car insurance, long-term care insurance, life insurance, Medicare, Medicaid, and any other insurance policy.

- ☐ Gather legal documents related to healthcare and possessions, such as a power of attorney, living will, trusts, or last will and testament.

- ☐ Gather information regarding your loved one's debt, including mortgages, loans, unpaid bills, credit cards, and other debt.

- ☐ Gather documents related to your loved one's admission to a healthcare facility.

- ☐ Find out if your loved one has legal responsibility for another individual, such as a spouse or an adult child with disabilities. What are the needs of this individual?

- ☐ Determine if and when your loved one may need full-time care assistance, either at home or in a long-term care facility. You may need to discuss this with your loved one's physician and other family members and friends who may help with your loved one's care.

- ☐ Discuss the likelihood of you and other primary caregivers becoming disabled and/or unable to care for your loved one.

- ☐ Determine who will care for your loved one if you are unable to do so.

- ☐ Gather information about all involved parties, including descendants, spouses, other family members, caregivers, financial planners, family attorneys, accountants, and others. You should be able to provide contact information for each individual.

- ☐ Ask the elder law attorney if there are other documents and information that you need to bring with you to the appointment, such as specific forms of identification.

Once you and your loved one have selected an elder law attorney and gathered the information you need for your first appointment, you will need to know what to discuss when you get to your appointment. The following checklist provides several important topics to discuss.

Checklist: Topics to discuss with your elder law attorney

☐ Discuss options for healthcare, including durable power of attorney for healthcare, living wills, and Do Not Resuscitate (DNR) orders.

☐ Discuss options for possessions, including durable power of attorney for finances, last will and testament, and living trusts.

☐ Discuss options for guardianship of minor children and adult children with disabilities, which should be included in guardianship documents (transfer guardianship before death) as well as in the last will and testament (transfer guardianship after death).

☐ Discuss options for financing care, including Medicare, Medicaid, insurance, veterans benefits, and Social Security.

☐ Discuss options for living arrangements, including long-term care or in-home care. (See *Home Care, Long-Term Care, Memory Care Units, and Other Living Arrangements* for more information.)

Once you have legal documents in place, you should review documents periodically to ensure that they still reflect your loved one's latest wishes. This review should happen as frequently as needed while your loved one is still legally competent to make changes to each document. The checklist below provides some important reasons to review legal documents. Note that although some of the reasons are listed under a specific document, they may apply to more than one document. In addition, documents should be reviewed after these circumstances, but they do not have to be changed unless your loved one deems it necessary.

Checklist: Reasons to review legal documents

Power of attorney:

☐ Your loved one is no longer legally qualified to be a power of attorney (also applies to executor of the will and trustees).

☐ The person listed as the power of attorney is no longer capable or willing to manage financial or healthcare decisions (also applies to executor of the will and trustees). This may happen if family tensions, health, or other circumstances cause too much stress for the individual.

- ☐ The person listed as the power of attorney consistently goes against your loved one's wishes or abuses their power.

- ☐ The person listed as the power of attorney no longer lives in close proximity to your loved one (either because they moved or because your loved one moved).

Living will and advance directives:

- ☐ Your loved one has a change in health or mental state.

- ☐ Your loved one's living arrangements change.

- ☐ Your loved one changes their mind about contents of the legal document (applies to all legal documents).

Last will and testament and living trust:

- ☐ Your loved one retires.

- ☐ Your loved one moves to a different state.

- ☐ There is a birth, adoption, or death in the family.

- ☐ There is a marriage or divorce in the family.

- ☐ There is a falling out or reconciliation between your loved one and another family member or friend.

- ☐ A minor child who is under your loved one's guardianship turns 18.

- ☐ Beneficiaries reach a milestone age or personal situation as stated by the will or trust (e.g., items in a trust may transfer to an individual at the age of 25, when they get married, etc.).

- ☐ Beneficiaries are added to or removed from accounts.

- ☐ Property or investments are bought or sold.

- ☐ Sources of income or debt change.

- ☐ Tax laws change.

- ☐ There is a substantial increase or decrease in your loved one's estate.

- ☐ There is a substantial change to a business owned by your loved one.

- ☐ A family member states a preference for inheriting a specific item, as long as the rest of the family is in agreement.

- ☐ A charity that interests your loved one opens, closes, or has a change in needs that your loved one wants to support.

Discussing Legal Documents

Creating legal documents as soon as possible, either before or after diagnosis, is the best way to ensure that your loved one's wishes will be followed when they become mentally incompetent or pass away. In order for your loved one to sign legal documents, they must be mentally competent, able to make rational decisions, and able to understand the contents of the documents and the legal ramifications of signing the documents. For individuals with dementia such as Alzheimer's disease, the earlier these documents are signed in the course of the disease, the more likely it is that the document will stand firm in a court of law.

If your loved one has been recently diagnosed with Alzheimer's disease and they do not have the recommended legal documents in place, you need to encourage your loved one to start thinking about and creating these documents. Some individuals may feel that this is the beginning of their loss of independence, and the realization that they can no longer be completely independent may be a source of contention for some families. People will react differently to these types of requests from loved ones.

In my friend Amy's case, her father was giving money away to scam artists and making questionable purchases on a limited income. Amy knew that she had to act soon or her parents would be in a worse position. Because her father refused to discuss legal documents with her, Amy asked her father's friends to convince her dad to relinquish control.

Amy needed a unique approach when talking to her father about legal documents. You may also find that you need to try several approaches before one works. The checklist below provides some ideas for how to start the discussion about legal documents with your loved one. Some of these ideas may be more appropriate for you and your loved one than others, so use the ones that seem most natural for you. Keep in mind that you may have to take control of your loved one's finances and legal matters against their wishes for their own good, perhaps even going to court to officially have them declared legally incompetent if that is what it takes.

Checklist: How to discuss legal documents with your loved one

- ☐ Ask permission to talk about end-of-life issues, because many people avoid this topic.

- ☐ Ask your loved one if they have considered what will happen to them and their possessions if they become incapacitated or die.

- ☐ Tell your loved one that you are in the process of making these legal documents for yourself, and encourage them to take steps to make these legal documents for themselves.

- ☐ Start with a story of someone else's experience of how they wished they would have had legal documents in place or they were thankful that they had such documents.

- ☐ Ask a close friend of your loved one or your loved one's minister to encourage them to get their affairs in order.

- ☐ Take notice of opportunities to open the conversation, such as the death of a loved one, a news story, medical checkups, family gatherings, movies, sermons, and so on. Follow through with the conversation about legal documents as opportunities appear.

- ☐ If you are the spouse, ask your loved one to discuss legal matters with you so you can make decisions together now rather than having to make them alone later.

- ☐ If you are the adult child, ask your parents and siblings to hold a family meeting (immediate family only) to discuss important legal matters. Turn it into a family project in which everyone creates their own legal documents.

- ☐ Make an "appointment" to discuss legal matters. Select an appropriate time and place for the discussion; usually a private place is best. Keep the discussion light and make an event of it.

- ☐ Mention to your loved one that talking about this earlier and more frequently will help you ensure that their wishes are being met in the future because you and other caregivers will understand how they would have chosen for themselves.

- ☐ Tell your loved one that having the discussion now will save a lot of pain and anxiety for caregivers later.

- ☐ Mention that your loved one's attorney or physician mentioned that it would be helpful to create legal documents related to finances and healthcare.

- ☐ Encourage your loved one to speak with their physician about medical options at the end of life so they understand the options they want to list in their legal documents.

- ☐ Start discussions early. It is more comfortable to talk about these topics when it is a hypothetical future issue rather than a current, looming one. For individuals with Alzheimer's disease, waiting too long could mean that they are no longer legally competent to make legal documents.

- ☐ Don't be surprised if you encounter resistance the first time you try. Don't be discouraged or force the issue. Come back to the discussion later when an opening presents itself.

- ☐ Allow your loved one to set the pace of the conversation.

- ☐ Make sure you are a good listener during the conversation. Listen for clues about your loved one's wishes, and don't turn it into a debate.

- ☐ Be caring and supportive, and don't be selfish or demanding.

- ☐ If your loved one is already making poor financial choices and refuses to sign legal documents, you may need to take them to court to have them declared legally incompetent in order to have a conservator or guardian appointed for them.

- ☐ If your loved one already has legal documents in place, ask them to review the documents to make sure they still reflect their wishes in light of their new diagnosis.

- ☐ Make sure your loved one knows you want to have this discussion because you care about them.

Starting the discussion about legal documents is perhaps the most uncomfortable part of the entire process. Once your loved one has accepted the fact that legal documents need to be created, the process of making the documents can be tedious but also rewarding and comforting. The most important documents to create are the durable power of attorney for healthcare and durable power of attorney for finances. Once these documents are in place, you and your loved one can focus on creating a living will and other advance directives as well as creating a last will and testament and living trust, if desired.

Legal Documents for Healthcare

Your loved one's need for good healthcare will grow as they progress through Alzheimer's disease. (See *Dementia, Alzheimer's Disease Stages, Treatment Options, and Other Medical Considerations* for more information.) However, at some point in the course of the disease, your loved one will be unable to make their own healthcare choices, either because they cannot understand their medical choices, they cannot rationally make a decision, or they are unable to communicate their wishes. Therefore, having legal documents related to their healthcare wishes is vital to them receiving the care they would have chosen for themselves. Legal documents related to healthcare include a durable power of attorney for healthcare, living will, and other advance directives.

Durable Power of Attorney for Healthcare

A durable power of attorney for healthcare is created to name a single individual or group of individuals who will be allowed to make healthcare decisions for your loved one. A durable power of attorney for healthcare is called "durable" because it is active both before and after the principal is declared mentally incompetent. Choosing a good healthcare agent is one of the most important legal decisions your loved one will make. See the checklists below for important aspects to consider when creating a durable power of attorney for healthcare.

Checklist: Basics about a durable power of attorney for healthcare

☐ The durable power of attorney for healthcare document may also be called a healthcare power of attorney, medical power of attorney, appointment of a healthcare agent, or healthcare proxy.

☐ The individual creating the durable power of attorney for healthcare is called the principal. In this book, your loved one with Alzheimer's disease is assumed to be the principal.

☐ The individual named to make healthcare decisions for the principal is called the healthcare agent. They may also be called a surrogate, attorney-in-fact, healthcare representative, or healthcare proxy.

☐ The healthcare agent is only allowed to make medical decisions, not financial decisions, for your loved one.

☐ The durable power of attorney for healthcare is valid for both temporary (e.g., after an accident) and permanent (e.g., late-stage Alzheimer's disease) incapacitation.

☐ Although the durable power of attorney for healthcare is valid as soon as it is signed, physicians usually do not take advice from the healthcare agent as long as your loved one is capable of making decisions.

☐ The durable power of attorney for healthcare can be revoked or changed at any time, as long as your loved one is still legally competent.

☐ Your loved one should include a HIPAA release in the durable power of attorney for healthcare so the healthcare agent can access your loved one's medical records.

☐ A major benefit to having a healthcare agent compared to only a living will is that the healthcare agent can make all healthcare decisions in real time based on current information, whereas the living will is designed for a limited number of hypothetical situations.

☐ If your loved one becomes incapacitated and does not have a healthcare agent, they will either be appointed a healthcare proxy by a physician (a short-term solution) or will need a guardian appointed by the court (a long-term solution).

Checklist: Responsibilities of the principal

☐ Determine if there are any state laws restricting the choice of healthcare agent. For example, does the healthcare agent have to be a resident of the same state as your loved one?

☐ Choose a healthcare agent based on desired characteristics of a healthcare agent. Make sure the chosen agent is willing to accept this responsibility. Some states require that only one healthcare agent has power at a time, but some allow multiple agents.

☐ If more than one healthcare agent is chosen to act at the same time, all agents must be present and agree on medical actions before medical personnel will act on the decisions. This makes it complicated for physicians to act, especially if the agents do not agree.

☐ Choose an alternative healthcare agent if the original healthcare agent is unavailable or is unwilling to serve.

☐ Stipulate any restrictions on the healthcare agent, such as when the agent can make decisions (e.g., after diagnosis of a terminal illness, when the principal is permanently unconscious, etc.).

☐ Name any individuals who should *not* have any role in making healthcare decisions. This may be an estranged family member or in-laws.

☐ Create and sign the durable power of attorney for healthcare document. If your loved one spends significant time in more than one state, a durable power of attorney for healthcare document should be created for each state.

☐ Distribute copies of the durable power of attorney for healthcare to regular healthcare providers, the local hospital, the healthcare agent and alternative healthcare agent, and close family members.

☐ Keep a copy of the durable power of attorney document in an easily accessible place at home, and tell the healthcare agent and close family members where to find the document.

☐ Discuss responsibilities of the healthcare agent and any advance directives with the chosen agent(s).

☐ Discuss with the healthcare agent any values and beliefs that would affect healthcare decisions. Examples are religious beliefs that would dictate refusal of medical treatments, aspects that give your loved one's life meaning (family, career, independence, etc.), concerns about death or dying, and financial concerns.

☐ Tell family members whom the chosen healthcare agent is and why.

☐ If one healthcare agent become unwilling or unable to serve, or if your loved one wishes to revoke the agent's power, your loved one will need to create a new document and destroy all old documents.

Checklist: Characteristics of a good healthcare agent

☐ Meets the state's legal requirements for healthcare agents, including being over the age of 18.

☐ Will likely be available until your loved one's death (i.e., not someone who is close to death or has a terminal illness).

☐ Has a close, amicable relationship with your loved one; someone your loved one trusts with their life.

☐ Willing to take on the role of healthcare agent.

☐ Understands the significance of the healthcare agent role.

☐ Willing to discuss sensitive issues with your loved one.

☐ Shares your loved one's views and values regarding life, death, and medical treatments.

- [ ] Willing to follow all the stipulations in the living will, even if the agent does not agree with the stipulations.

- [ ] Willing to stand firm in the face of adversity if others do not agree with your loved one's wishes.

- [ ] Lives in close proximity to your loved one and is available to attend doctor's appointments or could travel to be close by if needed.

- [ ] Flexible and able to stay calm under pressure.

- [ ] Level-headed and mature.

- [ ] Not afraid to ask questions of healthcare providers.

- [ ] Not easily intimidated or overwhelmed by medical jargon or information.

- [ ] Not someone your loved one picks out of guilt or obligation.

- [ ] Not someone who is your loved one's healthcare provider, a relative of a healthcare provider, an employee at a business or government agency that finances your loved one's care, or anyone else who may have a conflict of interest.

- [ ] Common choices include a spouse, life partner, adult child, sibling, or trusted friend.

If you are close to the individual with Alzheimer's disease, such as a spouse or adult child, you may be called upon to be their healthcare agent. If you are asked to take on this role, what responsibilities will you have? See the checklist below for some common responsibilities of a healthcare agent.

Checklist: Responsibilities of a healthcare agent

Before making healthcare decisions:

- [ ] Discuss healthcare preferences with your loved one, including wishes for life-sustaining treatments. This should include preferences listed in your loved one's living will.

- [ ] Understand your loved one's current medications, including dosing and scheduling, as well as any allergies.

☐ Make sure physicians and other healthcare personnel as well as close family members have the most recent copies of all healthcare-related legal documents, such as power of attorney, living will, and advance directives.

☐ Carry a copy of the durable power of attorney for healthcare with you to show to facilities in case they have misplaced the copy you gave them.

☐ Ensure that the power of attorney document will be accepted by clinics, hospitals, and healthcare providers.

☐ Make sure the medical staff understands that you are the healthcare agent.

Making decisions:

☐ Receive and understand information about your loved one's medical condition, including prognosis with and without treatment. Stay informed as your loved one's medical condition changes.

☐ Be present for support and consultation during medical tests and procedures.

☐ Access your loved one's medical records; because of HIPAA laws, the healthcare agent must present the durable power of attorney for healthcare document to be granted access to medical records.

☐ Discuss healthcare options with the medical team; understand the pros and cons of different options. Write down information as needed. (See *Dementia, Alzheimer's Disease Stages, Treatment Options, and Other Medical Considerations* for more information.)

☐ Write down questions to ask the physician, and ask them at the next opportunity. Prioritize more important questions first.

☐ Seek second opinions as needed.

☐ Get support from medical staff for decisions, including physicians, nurses, social workers, chaplains, members of the ethics committee, and others.

☐ Make healthcare decisions for your loved one; decisions should be similar to choices your loved one would make and in your loved one's best interest.

☐ After decisions have been made, pass the decisions on to healthcare workers and caregivers.

☐ Sign consent forms for medical procedures.

Types of decisions:

☐ Choose your loved one's physicians and other healthcare providers.

☐ Choose care facilities for your loved one.

☐ Approve a transfer of care between facilities or between physicians.

☐ Approve medical treatments that your loved one will receive, including but not limited to medications, therapy, and surgery.

☐ Withhold or withdraw medical treatments according to the living will or your loved one's religious or cultural views, such as withholding artificial nutrition and hydration or blood transfusions.

☐ Authorize or refuse participation in medical research; can also authorize that experimental treatments be stopped.

☐ Approve or revoke DNR or DNI (Do Not Intubate) orders after discussing the pros and cons with a physician.

☐ Choose whether your loved one will die at home or in a healthcare facility.

☐ Decide when to start or stop providing only palliative care, comfort care, or hospice care.

☐ Give consent for organ donation and autopsy; your loved one's preference for this may be in the living will.

Monitoring care:

☐ Know what medications your loved one takes, including doses and schedules. This includes prescription and over-the-counter medications as well as vitamins and supplements. Make sure your loved one takes medications as prescribed.

- ☐ Make sure all prescribed treatments, tests, and procedures are being performed as ordered by the physician.

- ☐ Know what treatments should be started or stopped when your loved one is transferred to a new location or facility.

- ☐ Make sure pain and other symptoms are well managed.

- ☐ Provide comfort care as needed and allowed, such as giving ice chips, walking, assisting to the bathroom, etc.

- ☐ Be an advocate for your loved one if healthcare providers are not being responsive to requests.

- ☐ Post out-of-hospital DNR forms in your loved one's home, if desired.

- ☐ Know what to do or who to contact in case of a medical emergency.

Other:

- ☐ Fill out applications or paperwork for long-term care facilities, hospital admission, doctor's appointments, etc.

- ☐ Inform the family about your loved one's condition.

- ☐ Mediate conflict between family members.

- ☐ Do whatever is needed to stay in touch with your emotions, including talking to a counselor or clergy member.

Advance Directives

Advance directives are legal healthcare documents that stipulate the actions your loved one wants physicians and other medical personnel to take during the course of their treatment. Some advance directives, such as the living will, can cover many situations and many healthcare actions. Other advance directives, such as the Do Not Resuscitate order, cover only one medical action in one specific circumstance. Usually no legal representative is named in an advance directive, but a healthcare agent or other healthcare representative should know and understand the contents of the advance directives put in place by your loved one. For more information about advance directives, see the Resources section at the end of the book.

Living Will

The living will is a document that provides instructions about your loved one's desires for life-prolonging medical actions during specific circumstances. For example, if your loved one is declining rapidly and has no quality of life, the living will may stipulate that your loved one does not want to be subjected to artificial nutrition and hydration in order to prolong life. The checklists below provide basic information about living wills.

Checklist: Basics about a living will

☐ Provides instructions for healthcare personnel about life-sustaining and other medical treatments.

☐ May also be called a directive to physicians, healthcare declaration, or medical directive.

☐ Can be completed without a lawyer in many states, although many states have specific rules about forms for advance directives.

☐ Most states have a witnessing requirement for the living will and other advance directives. Most states require two witnesses and/or a notary. Generally the person's healthcare agent, family members, and healthcare providers cannot be witnesses.

☐ Becomes valid as soon as it is signed and does not have an expiration date.

☐ Only becomes effective once your loved one is no longer mentally competent and once they are near the end of life. Different states may have different requirements for this effective date.

☐ Outlines when specific medical treatments should be administered, withdrawn, or withheld. Withholding medical treatment (i.e., never starting treatment) is often an easier decision for healthcare agents than withdrawing medical treatment (i.e., stopping treatment once it is started).

☐ Gives reassurance to the healthcare agent that they are following your wishes.

- ☐ Can be used to direct medical decisions if your healthcare agent is unavailable.

- ☐ Is essential for individuals who do not have anyone to be their healthcare agent.

- ☐ Cannot be used by a healthcare agent or family member to request the principal's medical records.

- ☐ Can be changed as many times as desired until the principal is no longer legally competent.

- ☐ Cannot be followed by emergency medical personnel who are called to a home or long-term care facility. They are only responsible for keeping the individual alive until they are transferred to a medical facility.

- ☐ Having a living will in combination with a durable power of attorney for healthcare provides the greatest certainty that your loved one's wishes for their medical care will be followed.

- ☐ If your loved one does not have a living will or other advance directives and is incapacitated, the healthcare agent, healthcare proxy, or guardian will need to make healthcare decisions without any input from your loved one.

Checklist: Medical treatments that may be covered in a living will

- ☐ Do Not Resuscitate (DNR) order

- ☐ Do Not Intubate (DNI) order

- ☐ Use of artificial nutrition and hydration

- ☐ Organ, tissue, and body donation

- ☐ Use of dialysis

- ☐ Use of aggressive treatments

- ☐ Options for a mental facility

- ☐ Palliative care

- ☐ Transfer to hospital

- ☐ Autopsy

Checklist: Responsibilities of the principal

☐ Use the correct living will form required by the state. An elder law attorney may be a good resource for this information. If your loved one spends significant time in more than one state, a living will should be completed for each state.

☐ Get information from a physician about the types of life-sustaining treatments that are available.

☐ Decide their preferences for advance directives such as Do Not Resuscitate forms, artificial nutrition and hydration, organ donation, and other medical treatments.

☐ Write the living will in such a way that it does not restrict the healthcare agent in ways that are not intended (such as stating that you never want to be placed on a ventilator).

☐ Create and sign the living will with the help of an attorney and witnesses.

☐ Store the living will in a safe but easily accessible location (NOT a safe deposit box), and tell the healthcare agent or other family members where the document is stored.

☐ Give regular healthcare providers, hospitals, the healthcare agent, family members, and other involved parties a copy of the living will.

☐ Discuss medical preferences listed in the living will with medical personnel, caregivers, the healthcare agent, and family members.

☐ Make sure chosen physicians will honor the instructions in the living will; if the physician refuses to honor some of your wishes, find a different physician who will.

Checklist: Situations to consider when deciding about life-prolonging medical procedures

Would my loved one want life-prolonging care if they:

☐ Could no longer interact with friends and loved ones?

☐ Could no longer think or talk clearly?

- ☐ Could no longer respond to demands or requests?

- ☐ Could no longer walk independently?

- ☐ Could no longer contribute to their family's well-being?

- ☐ Could no longer control bowel and bladder activity?

- ☐ Could no longer perform activities of daily living independently (e.g., eating, toileting, dressing, etc.)?

- ☐ Had advanced dementia and could no longer recognize loved ones?

- ☐ Had significant brain damage?

- ☐ Were confined to the house or bed?

- ☐ Were in constant discomfort (pain, nausea, etc.) that could not be controlled with medication?

- ☐ Were in a permanent coma?

- ☐ Were a severe emotional or financial burden on their family?

- ☐ Required dialysis to stay alive?

- ☐ Required artificial nutrition and hydration to survive?

- ☐ Required mechanical ventilation to survive?

If your loved one has stipulated circumstances in which they felt that life would no longer be worth living, they may provide instructions for when they would want their healthcare agent to sign a Do Not Resuscitate (DNR) or Do Not Intubate (DNI) order. Instructions for when to sign a DNR order are one of the most common items included in a living will.

Do Not Resuscitate (DNR) and Do Not Intubate (DNI) Orders

Unless your loved one has a DNR order, medical personnel are legally and ethically required to perform heroic efforts to bring your loved one back to life if they undergo cardiac or respiratory arrest. In the absence of a DNR order, not using heroic efforts in these circumstances could instigate a court hearing and potential removal of their medical license. With a DNR order, however, medical personnel could also be liable for legal action if they *do* perform heroic efforts to bring the individual back to life, although most courts will not prosecute medical staff, especially emergency personnel, for performing cardiopulmonary resuscitation (CPR) if they were unaware of the DNR order.

Your loved one's wishes for a DNR or DNI order may be stated in the living will, but the actual DNR and DNI orders require a separate legal document. The checklist below provides details about DNR and DNI orders.

Checklist: Basics about DNR and DNI orders

- [ ] If your loved one has a DNR order, physicians and other medical personnel will not use heroic efforts to bring your loved one back to life if they undergo cardiac arrest (the heart stops beating) or respiratory arrest (your loved one stops breathing). This primarily refers to administration of CPR but may also refer to mechanical ventilation (using a machine to breathe for your loved one) and the use of a defibrillator (a machine that produces an electric shock to start the heart beating again).

- [ ] A DNR order is *not* an order not to treat the patient. It simply withholds CPR. Other treatments, such as pain medication, antibiotics, comfort care measures, and even aggressive treatment of a disease can all still be given when a DNR order is in effect.

- [ ] A DNR order may also be called an Allow Natural Death (AND) form in some states.

- [ ] If your loved one has a DNI order, physicians and other medical personnel will not intubate your loved one. Intubation involves putting a tube down the throat to aid in breathing or to hook up mechanical ventilation/artificial breathing.

- [ ] A DNR or DNI order can be requested by your loved one or your loved one's healthcare agent, but the order *must* be signed by a physician.

- [ ] A DNR or DNI order can be signed or revoked at any time.

- [ ] Medical personnel must have a signed DNR or DNI order in their medical records for it to be honored.

- ☐ If your loved one is in the hospital, the DNR or DNI order should be prominently displayed by your loved one's bed. If it is not, make sure the medical staff has a copy of the DNR or DNI order and ask them to post a copy in your loved one's room.

- ☐ A DNR order is only effective in a hospital or doctor's office. If your loved one is seriously ill and wants a DNR order at home where emergency medical personnel may provide care, they will need an out-of-hospital DNR order posted in their home; this may be on an official form, wallet card, or bracelet.

- ☐ If an out-of-hospital DNR order is not obviously posted, emergency medical personnel and bystanders will not be held legally responsible if they perform CPR on your loved one.

Signing a DNR order is a significant step and should not be taken lightly. The checklists below provide some common reasons to sign, not sign, or revoke a DNR order. Remember that each individual's circumstances are different, so you may not want to sign a DNR for your loved one under all of these circumstances. In addition, there may be other circumstances not listed that may provide sufficient reason to sign (or not sign) a DNR order.

Checklist: When should my loved one have a DNR order?

- ☐ If they are likely a few days or hours away from death.

- ☐ If they are frail and CPR may cause more damage (e.g., broken ribs) than good.

- ☐ If they are in a permanent coma with little or no chance of recovery.

- ☐ If the individual has little chance of leaving the hospital even if successfully revived.

- ☐ If successful CPR has little chance of helping the individual recover for more than a few days.

- ☐ If they have a low quality of life and medical treatments are unlikely to restore quality of life, such as with very late-stage Alzheimer's disease.

- ☐ If they are bed-bound and have lost the ability to swallow (e.g., they cannot consume food or drink through the mouth).

- ☐ If they are in substantial pain due to a terminal condition that is not relieved by pain medication.

- ☐ If they are on mechanical ventilation with no chance of recovery.

- ☐ If they are in multi-organ failure (kidney, liver, heart, etc.).

- ☐ If a physician states that they would recommend a DNR order.

- ☐ Under any circumstances stated in the living will. Your loved one should consider circumstances under which they would or would not want a DNR order signed, including circumstances listed in these checklists, and record their wishes in their living will.

Checklist: When should my loved one NOT have a DNR order?

- ☐ If they are going into surgery. (Active DNR orders are often suspended for the duration of the surgery.)

- ☐ If they recover from a life-threatening illness or disease.

- ☐ If they are months or years away from death.

- ☐ If they have a good chance of recovery after treatment.

- ☐ If successful CPR will allow the individual to leave the hospital and regain some quality of life.

The choice of whether to approve a DNR order is a major decision that will likely be one of the hardest you have to make as a healthcare agent. However, if your loved one has reached a stage of disease in which they are close to death and have no chance of recovery, a DNR order may save them from a prolonged, painful dying process. If your loved one has given stipulations for the use of a DNR or DNI order in their living will, those orders should be followed explicitly. Although it is hard to lose a loved one, sometimes the best thing you can do for them is let them die naturally if they are already near death.

Artificial Nutrition and Hydration

Artificial nutrition and hydration are primarily used when your loved one is no longer able to swallow enough food and water to maintain adequate nutritional intake. Individuals with Alzheimer's disease often lose the ability to swallow properly, and swallowing often leads to aspiration, or the intake of food or liquid into the lungs. This can lead to infections, particularly pneumonia, which can be fatal in frail, elderly individuals. In fact, aspiration pneumonia is the leading cause of death for individuals with Alzheimer's disease. For individuals who are unable to swallow properly, artificial nutrition and hydration may be required to sustain life and prevent infection. To learn more about artificial nutrition and hydration, see the checklist below.

Checklist: Basics about artificial nutrition and hydration

- ☐ There are two categories of artificial nutrition and hydration: parenteral and enteral.

- ☐ Parenteral nutrition is nutrition that is administered directly into the veins via an intravenous (IV) tube.

- ☐ Parenteral nutrition is often used to administer hydration (water) and electrolytes (sodium, calcium, chloride, magnesium, potassium, etc.).

- ☐ Enteral nutrition is nutrition that is administered directly into the stomach via a small tube inserted through the nose (short-term) or through an incision in the abdominal cavity (long-term).

- ☐ Enteral nutrition is often used to administer calories via a liquid formula that contains proteins, carbohydrates, and fats. The required caloric content and nutritional makeup of the formula is chosen based on the individual's needs.

- ☐ Your loved one's living will can state when nutrition should be administered, when it should be withheld, and when it should be withdrawn.

- ☐ Common reasons to administer artificial nutrition and hydration include temporarily controlling what enters the stomach (such as after surgery or to help heal stomach ulcers) or providing a source of nutrition for individuals who cannot swallow (such as some Alzheimer's patients and quadriplegics).

☐ Artificial nutrition and hydration are often withheld or withdrawn if the individual is close to death and the nutrition will not help them recover or give them a better quality of life.

☐ Experts agree that for individuals who are close to death, withholding nutrition and hydration does not cause pain or feelings of hunger or thirst.

☐ Experts also agree that for frail individuals near the end of life, providing nutrition and hydration may cause more harm than good because it puts stress on failing kidneys and digestive system.

☐ Individuals who are close to death who do not receive artificial nutrition and hydration may live as long as two weeks or more before death, but they may also pass away within a day or two, depending on their physical state.

Organ, Tissue, and Body Donation

Some individuals would like their healthy organs or tissues donated to others who need them, and some individuals choose to have their entire body donated for medical research or medical teaching. If your loved one would like to donate their organs, tissues, or body, the checklist below provides some important information for your loved one to consider. For more information about organ donation, see websites listed in the Resources section at the back of the book.

Checklist: Basics about organ, tissue, and body donation

☐ The living will can state whether your loved one wants their healthy organs and/or tissues donated to others who may benefit from them. This can also be stated on your driver's license in many states.

☐ Commonly donated organs include the heart, liver, kidneys, lungs, pancreas, eyes, and intestines.

☐ Commonly donated tissues include the cornea, skin, heart valves, blood vessels, bones, and tendons.

□ In order to donate organs, the organs must receive blood until they can be harvested. Therefore, your loved one may need to be put on mechanical ventilation until the harvesting procedure is complete, even if they had a DNI order. The living will should state that your loved one understands the need for this temporary intervention.

□ The living will can also state if your loved one wants their body donated for research or to a medical teaching facility for students.

□ If your loved one wants to donate their body, their will must state where they want their body donated, and they need to make arrangements with the facility before their death. In addition, many institutions require a fee for accepting a donated body due to lack of funding.

□ Donation of organs, tissues, or body usually means that an autopsy would not be beneficial for your loved one, although individuals with Alzheimer's disease may specifically have only their brain autopsied to identify characteristic lesions associated with Alzheimer's disease.

□ Some individuals who are old or terminally ill may not have organs that are suitable for donation.

□ Even if their organs are harvested, your loved one's body can still be shown at the funeral.

Other Medical Directives

Many other medical directives can be given in a living will, and a living will can be changed to reflect your loved one's diagnosis of Alzheimer's disease, provided your loved one makes the changes while they are still legally competent. The checklist below provides descriptions of a few less-common medical directives.

Checklist: Basics about less-common medical directives

□ **Dialysis.** Dialysis is used to remove toxins from the blood when the kidneys no longer work properly. Dialysis is usually performed at least three times per week for individuals with minimal kidney function, and it often takes 3–4 hours for each session, leaving the individual exhausted. Individuals on frequent dialysis usually have a fistula or shunt to ease access to the blood vessels for dialysis. If not cared for properly, these access points can become infected. However, many individuals are on dialysis for years with minimal complications. Without dialysis, individuals with failing kidneys will die quickly from too many toxins in the blood.

☐ **Medical treatments.** Some individuals with progressive Alzheimer's disease may choose to not receive aggressive treatments such as radiation or chemotherapy after a cancer diagnosis or even antibiotics after being diagnosed with an infection. These treatments may cause your loved one's physical or mental state to worsen, or it could prolong their life when the quality of life is already low.

☐ **Care facilities.** Individuals with Alzheimer's disease slowly lose their mental capabilities, often leaving them depressed, violent, or suicidal. Some individuals with Alzheimer's disease stipulate in their living will when they would be willing to be admitted to a mental or long-term care facility and which facility they would choose to be admitted to.

☐ **Palliative care.** Many individuals with Alzheimer's disease may opt to receive only palliative care in the advanced stages of the disease. *Palliative care* refers to care that only relieves suffering and provides comfort measures such as pain medication or medication to relieve constipation. Palliative care does NOT provide other medical treatments such as antibiotics and artificial nutrition and hydration. It is used primarily to maintain your loved one's dignity and quality of life until their natural death. Palliative care is often given at home through hospice care. For more information about palliative and hospice care, see the Resources section at the end of the book.

☐ **Transfer to hospital.** If given a choice, most individuals state that they would rather die at home than in a hospital. Therefore, some individuals state in their living will that they do not want to be transferred to a hospital when they are near death, or they state the circumstances under which they would choose to go to a hospital. For individuals with Alzheimer's disease, transferring locations may cause confusion and hasten death, so in the late stages of the disease they should not be moved to a new location, even if it is their own home, unless it is medically necessary.

☐ **Autopsy.** The only way to definitively diagnose Alzheimer's disease is to do a brain autopsy after death to identify characteristic brain lesions associated with Alzheimer's disease. Some individuals may choose to state in their living will or in their last will and testament whether they would like to have an autopsy performed after their death. Note that the cost of an autopsy is often charged to the patient if it is elective.

Physician Orders for Life-Sustaining Treatment (POLST)

Many of the advance directives summarized here can be stated in a simple form called a Physician Orders for Life-Sustaining Treatment, or POLST (also called MOLST, medical orders for life-sustaining treatment). The POLST form is usually filled out in the presence of the physician or other qualified medical personnel as well as your loved one or your loved one's legal representative. The POLST form is then posted by your loved one's bed, usually on a brightly colored piece of paper, so that all medical personnel involved in your loved one's treatment are aware of the form and your loved one's choices for treatment.

The POLST form contains instructions from your loved one or your loved one's legal representative regarding end-of-life care, including use of CPR, artificial nutrition, and other medical interventions. The POLST form can also indicate the presence of an advance directive or living will document. Instructions given on the POLST form are regarded as direct physician orders and must be followed by all medical personnel. For more information about POLST, see the Resources section at the end of the book.

Legal Documents for Finances

In addition to being unable to make healthcare decisions, your loved one with Alzheimer's disease will likely be unable to make good financial decisions as they progress through the disease. This is because they are unable to understand basic financial concepts, recognize poor financial decisions and scams, and remember to pay bills. Therefore, choosing someone who can handle their financial affairs both during their lifetime and after their death will be vital to their financial stability. Your loved one can help ensure their finances will remain in good hands by establishing a durable power of attorney for finances, as well as by creating a last will and testament and perhaps a trust.

Durable Power of Attorney for Finances

A durable power of attorney for finances is created to name a single individual or group of individuals who will be allowed to make financial decisions for your loved one. Although likely not as important as choosing a good healthcare agent, choosing a qualified individual to make financial decisions is important for making sure your loved one's financial needs are taken care of while they are still alive. See the checklists below for important information about the durable power of attorney for finances.

Checklist: Basics about a durable power of attorney for finances

☐ The individual creating the durable power of attorney for finances is called the *principal*. In this book, your loved one with Alzheimer's disease is assumed to be the principal.

☐ The individual named to make financial decisions for the principal is called the *attorney-in-fact*.

☐ The attorney-in-fact is only allowed to make financial decisions, not healthcare decisions, for your loved one.

☐ The durable power of attorney for finances is valid as soon as it is signed, but the attorney-in-fact usually does not have any responsibilities before your loved one becomes legal incompetent except for specific duties stated in the document.

☐ The durable power of attorney for finances is valid for both individual transactions (e.g., selling a specific piece of property as designated in the document) and for global management of finances (e.g., after the principal is incapacitated).

☐ The durable power of attorney for finances can be revoked or changed at any time, as long as your loved one is still legally competent.

☐ The durable power of attorney for finances document will *not* allow the attorney-in-fact to obtain your loved one's medical records.

☐ If your loved one does not have an attorney-in-fact and becomes incapacitated, you or another individual will need to petition the court for conservatorship.

Checklist: Responsibilities of the principal

☐ Determine if there are any state laws restricting the choice of attorney-in-fact.

☐ Choose an attorney-in-fact based on desired characteristics of an attorney-in-fact. Make sure the chosen agent is willing to accept this responsibility. Usually having only one active attorney-in-fact at a time is best, because it eliminates disagreements about property.

☐ Choose an alternative attorney-in-fact if the original attorney-in-fact is unavailable or is unwilling to serve.

☐ Stipulate any restrictions on the attorney-in-fact, such as when the agent can make decisions (e.g., after the principal is legally incompetent) or which specific transactions the attorney-in-fact is responsible for.

☐ Create and sign the durable power of attorney for finances document.

☐ Distribute copies of the durable power of attorney for finances to banks, investment companies, insurance companies, utility companies, and other companies that your loved one interacts with financially.

☐ Keep a copy of the durable power of attorney for finances document in an easily accessible place at home, and tell the attorney-in-fact and close family members where to find the document.

☐ Discuss financial responsibilities, duties, and wishes with the attorney-in-fact.

☐ Discuss living trusts and last will and testament with the chosen agent(s), even if they are not the executor of the will or the trustee.

☐ Tell family members whom the chosen attorney-in-fact is and why.

☐ If one attorney-in-fact becomes unwilling or unable to serve, or if your loved one wishes to revoke the agent's power, your loved one will need to create a new document and destroy all old documents.

Checklist: Characteristics of a good attorney-in-fact

☐ Meets the state's legal requirements for an attorney-in-fact, including being over the age of 18.

- ☐ Has a close, amicable relationship with your loved one.

- ☐ Is willing to take on the role of attorney-in-fact.

- ☐ Lives in close proximity to your loved one.

- ☐ Is knowledgeable about financial matters and keeps good financial records.

- ☐ Is financially responsible, which will ensure that your loved one's bills are paid on time.

- ☐ Understands your loved one's goals and wishes for their finances.

- ☐ Understands your loved one's financial portfolio and knows where important financial documents are kept.

- ☐ Is trusted by close family members.

- ☐ If your loved one is married, they will likely choose their spouse as their attorney-in-fact.

- ☐ Other common options for attorney-in-fact are an adult child, sibling, trusted friend, family lawyer, or bank.

- ☐ Although it is possible to name more than one individual as the attorney-in-fact, usually it is best to name only one person in case there is conflict when making financial decisions.

- ☐ If the family is likely to have arguments over financial decisions and assets, using a neutral third party as the attorney-in-fact is often the best choice.

Checklist: Responsibilities of an attorney-in-fact

- ☐ Manage finances while your loved one is still living; after death, financial decisions and distribution of property fall to the executor of the will.

- ☐ Read the directions given in the durable power of attorney document and follow what it says.

- ☐ Make sure all relevant parties (banks, utility companies, investment brokers, insurance companies, etc.) have a copy of the durable power of attorney for finances.

☐ Ensure that the power of attorney document will be accepted by banks, utility companies, and other financial institutions.

☐ Make decisions that are in the best interest of your loved one, not the attorney-in-fact or your loved one's family members.

☐ Discuss financial goals and priorities with your loved one.

☐ Make sure that your loved one's financial needs are being met.

☐ Find out whether your loved one is eligible for financial services, including pensions, disability, Social Security, Medicare, Medicaid, veterans benefits, housing assistance, or food stamps (SNAP); then help your loved one apply for these services and benefits as appropriate. (For a benefits checkup website, see the Resources section at the end of the book.)

☐ Fill out reports required for government benefits such as Social Security income, veterans benefits, and disability income.

☐ Get legal advice about Medicaid eligibility from an elder law attorney.

☐ Involve your loved one in financial decisions for as long as possible.

☐ Research your loved one's past financial decisions to determine how they would have acted under different circumstances.

☐ Use common sense when making financial decisions for your loved one.

☐ Oversee bank accounts and balance checkbooks; make sure bank accounts are receiving interest and have no or low fees.

☐ Keep accurate and honest financial records.

☐ Pay bills, taxes, and other expenses on time.

☐ Purchase or sell property.

☐ Collect rent or unpaid debt.

☐ Keep real estate in good condition.

☐ Make investments carefully.

☐ Purchase insurance as needed, and cancel any unnecessary insurance policies.

- ☐ Keep your loved one's property safe through use of a safe deposit box, insurance, a security system, locks, and other safety measures.

- ☐ Keep their financial holdings separate from your loved one's financial holdings.

- ☐ Avoid conflicts of interest (i.e., situations in which a decision may benefit one party but harm your loved one).

- ☐ Resist borrowing or spending money for their own purposes or loaning money to others from your loved one's estate. Note that it is very easy for an attorney-in-fact to drain your loved one's financial resources because they have complete control of your loved one's accounts. Steps should be taken to prevent this.

- ☐ Give money away only if it is within your loved one's normal pattern of giving (e.g., birthday gifts for grandchildren, annual donations to charity, etc.).

- ☐ Not charge a fee for financial management services, unless the power of attorney document permits it.

- ☐ Be aware of financial abuse or scams that your loved one may be subject to.

Last Will and Testament

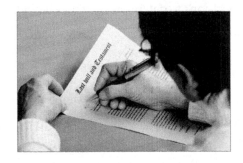

In contrast to a durable power of attorney for finances that names someone to manage property before your loved one's death, the last will and testament states how property should be distributed after your loved one's death. While not every possession needs to be listed individually in the will, large items or items with great sentimental value should be specifically designated for distribution. The checklists below provide some basics about the last will and testament as well as common items listed in the will and how they are frequently distributed. Remember that this list may not be inclusive, and ideas for distribution are examples only.

Checklist: Basics about a last will and testament

- ☐ The last will and testament, or will, provides instructions for how an individual wants their estate distributed after their death.

- [ ] The person writing the will is called the *testator*. After death, they are referred to as the *decedent*. In this book, your loved one with Alzheimer's disease is assumed to be the testator.

- [ ] The individual named to distribute property as listed in the will is called the *executor of the will*. The executor is usually a spouse, adult child, or family lawyer.

- [ ] Individuals who will receive property listed in the will are called *beneficiaries*. Beneficiaries are usually your loved one's spouse, children, grandchildren, siblings, friends, and favorite charities.

- [ ] Your loved one must be legally competent to write a valid will, and they must be over the age of 18.

- [ ] For the courts to recognize a will as valid, it must be written (as opposed to verbal) and contain at least two witness signatures.

- [ ] The will is only valid after your loved one's death.

- [ ] The will can be revoked or changed at any time, as long as your loved one is still legally competent.

- [ ] An amendment to the will can also be written; this is called a *codicil*.

- [ ] Your loved one's significant assets should be listed in the will *unless* beneficiaries are stated directly on an account (such as a savings account or insurance policy).

- [ ] Your loved one may be able to make a simple will (limited property and few beneficiaries) online or with purchased computer software, but complicated wills (a large estate with many beneficiaries) should be created with the help of a lawyer.

- [ ] In order for property to be distributed, the will must be filed with the probate court, which is the legal system that handles property distribution after someone's death. Most wills will not ever appear in court; if written well, the executor will be allowed to distribute your loved one's property out of court.

- [ ] If the will is not written or witnessed properly, if someone contests the will, or if your loved one does not have a will, the will may go through a lengthy probate process. In these circumstances, probate court can be expensive and time-consuming.

☐ Any documents that go through probate court, such as a will, become public record. Therefore, anyone can read the contents of the will and beneficiaries. To avoid probate court, a living trust can be created.

☐ Even if a living trust exists, everyone should have a will to distribute property not listed in the trust, including guardianship of minor children and distribution of personal items such as clothing and furniture.

☐ If your loved one dies without a will, the court will appoint an administrator of the estate to handle the distribution of property.

Checklist: Responsibilities of the testator

☐ Choose an executor of the will based on desired characteristics of an executor. Make sure the chosen executor is willing to accept this responsibility.

☐ Choose an alternative executor if the original executor is unavailable or is unwilling to serve.

☐ Determine which items should be listed in the will, and name beneficiaries for each item. Use specific names of beneficiaries rather than broad categories, such as "nieces and nephews."

☐ Choose alternate beneficiaries if the original beneficiary cannot accept the assets.

☐ Create and sign the last will and testament. State clearly in the document that this is a will.

☐ Distribute copies of the last will and testament to interested parties, including the executor, key family members, and a family lawyer.

☐ Keep a copy of the last will and testament in an easily accessible place at home, and tell the executor and close family members where to find the document.

☐ Discuss the distribution of property with the executor.

☐ If the primary executor becomes unwilling or unable to serve, or if your loved one wishes to change executors or change stipulations in the will, your loved one will need to create a new document and destroy all old documents.

☐ Review the will whenever there is a major change in your loved one's circumstances, such as a birth, death, marriage, or divorce in the family.

Checklist: Items commonly listed in the will

☐ **Guardianship for minor children.** One of the most important statements in a will is who will be the guardian of any minor children still in the household. Each child should have an individual or couple named as a guardian, even if the same individual or couple is named for every child. Common choices for guardianship of minor children include a surviving parent, grandparent, aunt or uncle, godparent, or trusted friend. Be sure to discuss this choice with the chosen guardian.

☐ **Guardianship for adult children with disabilities.** Similar to minor children, the will needs to state who will become guardian of an adult child with a disability. Similar options for guardianship are available as for minor children. However, because of the disability, some individuals may decline guardianship, so confirm that the individual is willing to become guardian before adding their name to the will.

☐ **Pets.** Although not as vital as naming a guardian for children, the will should also contain instructions for who should care for any pets that remain after your loved one's death. For most individuals, this will be a cat or dog, but it may also include animals such as horses, cattle, sheep, goats, snakes, mice, gerbils, birds, and other less common pets or farm animals.

☐ **Real estate, such as a primary residence, vacation home, or rental property.** If your loved one is married, real estate, especially a primary residence, is often passed to the surviving spouse. If no surviving spouse remains, real estate frequently goes to the oldest child or is sold and the proceeds split evenly between children.

☐ **Vehicles.** Vehicles such as cars, trucks, boats, RVs, ATVs, and others may be left to the surviving spouse, a child or grandchild who needs transportation (e.g., a grandchild going to college), or an individual who shares a similar hobby (e.g., a boat could be given to a son who shares a love of fishing); donated to a local charity; or sold and the proceeds divided among heirs.

☐ **Cash.** Cash is one of the most versatile possessions to pass on. First, available cash should be used to pay any debts or outstanding bills. Once debts are paid, cash can be distributed to family, friends, charities, or other organizations. Note that individuals who are listed as beneficiaries or joint owners of cash accounts such as checking or savings accounts usually have priority over any distribution listed in the will.

☐ **Investments.** Investments such as stocks, bonds, and mutual funds are often passed down to the surviving spouse, children, grandchildren, or siblings. They can also be gifted to some charities. Some investments allow you to list a beneficiary. If a beneficiary is listed on the investment, the investment does not need to be listed in the will.

☐ **Insurance payouts.** Insurance policies such as life insurance have a payout upon the policy holder's death. Most insurance policies that pay benefits on death will require you to list a beneficiary on the policy itself. However, if a beneficiary is not listed, the policy benefits can be distributed through the will. Common beneficiaries include a surviving spouse, children, or grandchildren.

☐ **Jewelry.** Jewelry, especially expensive or heirloom jewelry, should be included in the will to prevent family arguments. Wedding rings are often willed to the oldest daughter or granddaughter. A father's watch may go to the oldest son. Some family members may state a preference for receiving a specific piece of jewelry. Jewelry can also be sold and the proceeds distributed to the family members or donated to a charity.

☐ **Furniture.** If furniture is expensive or handmade, specific individuals in the family may want to take possession of those items. Basic furniture could be given to grandchildren who are just starting their own homes or donated to a local charity for families in need.

☐ **Household items.** Unless someone needs or wants a specific household item, common household items are often donated to a local charity or sold in an estate sale.

☐ **Clothing.** Most clothing items are donated to a local charity or given to someone who requests specific clothing items. A wedding dress may be passed down to a daughter or granddaughter.

☐ **Tools.** Tools may be passed on to children or grandchildren who need them. Unwanted tools may be donated to a local charity or sold in an estate sale.

☐ **Ownership in a business.** If your loved one owns a family business, the will can name the individual(s) who will take over your loved one's ownership shares and responsibilities. The transfer of responsibility will likely take place before your loved one's death. However, ownership shares in the business may be passed on before or after death. Ownership shares are often transferred to the individual who took over the business or split between surviving children.

☐ **Trusts.** If desired, a will can be used to set up a testamentary trust for managing your loved one's money after their death. This is common if the beneficiaries are still minors (under 18 years old) at the time of your loved one's death.

☐ **Funeral and burial arrangements.** If your loved one has purchased a burial plot or has specific instructions about the use of a particular funeral home, church, order of service, or headstone engraving, they should be included in the will and discussed with family members.

☐ **Other.** Other items of monetary or sentimental significance should be included in the will as well. These items can be willed to a specific individual or charity or they can be sold at an estate sale.

Individuals who have a last will and testament should also name an executor of their will in the will document as well as a successor executor in case the original executor becomes incapacitated. Characteristics of a good executor and responsibilities of an executor are listed in the checklists below.

Checklist: Characteristics of a good executor of the will

☐ Meets the state's legal requirements for executor, including being over the age of 18 with no prior felony convictions.

☐ Is a trusted individual, such as a spouse, adult child, family lawyer, or close friend, or a bank.

☐ Is willing to be executor of the will.

☐ Has the time and skills needed to properly execute the will.

☐ Is organized and meticulous when dealing with important documents.

Checklist: Responsibilities of an executor of the will

☐ Oversee the distribution of your loved one's property according to the will. The executor of the will has no legal authority while your loved one is still alive.

☐ Contact beneficiaries to attend a reading of the will.

☐ Consult with an attorney to help with the probate process.

☐ File legal documents in probate court to receive an official executor document that allows them to distribute the estate.

☐ Attend court appearances related to your loved one's will, if needed.

☐ Advocate with the court to have your loved one's assets distributed according to the will.

☐ Settle debts owed by your loved one, and collect on debts owed to your loved one.

☐ Appraise the value of your loved one's assets.

☐ File paperwork related to transferring property from your loved one to beneficiaries.

☐ Oversee the sale of real estate or other assets as listed in the will.

☐ Oversee an estate sale or donation of items to charity.

☐ File estate and other taxes for the decedent as necessary.

Trusts

In addition to a last will and testament, property can be transferred to beneficiaries through a trust. Trusts can seem very complicated at first, but they help shelter your loved one's assets and protect certain assets from taxes if executed correctly. Before forming a trust, talk to a financial planner, lawyer, or trust department at your local bank to help decide which type of trust will be best for your loved one. The checklists below include several facts about trusts.

Checklist: Terms related to trusts

☐ **Trust.** A document that creates an agreement between a grantor, trustee, and beneficiaries for how the grantor's property will be distributed to beneficiaries either during the grantor's lifetime or after the grantor's death.

☐ **Grantor.** The *grantor* is the person who creates the trust. The grantor may also be called the *trustor*, *settler*, or *donor*. In this book, your loved one with Alzheimer's disease is assumed to be the grantor.

☐ **Trustee.** The *trustee* is the person who manages the trust. The grantor is often named the trustee. The trustee can also be a spouse, adult child, family lawyer, or friend. Often a neutral third party such as a trust department at a bank will be named trustee. Successor trustees should also be named in case the primary trustee is unable to complete their duties.

☐ **Decedent.** The grantor after their death.

☐ **Beneficiary.** The individuals or other parties that receive property through the trust. Beneficiaries are usually the grantor's spouse, children, grandchildren, or friends. Beneficiaries can also be charitable organizations.

☐ **Property.** The items that are placed in the trust. The property in the trust may also be called the principal.

☐ **Surviving spouse.** The spouse of the grantor that is still alive after the grantor's death.

Checklist: Types of trusts

☐ **Living trust.** A living trust is a trust that is created and managed during your loved one's lifetime. Your loved one usually retains control of a living trust (i.e., they are the trustee) during their lifetime as long as they are mentally competent. Property in a living trust can be transferred to beneficiaries both while your loved one is still alive and after your loved one's death, depending on the stipulations in the trust. Because a living trust is a legal document describing how property in the trust is to be distributed, it does not have to go through probate court. This is the most common type of trust and the most advantageous for individuals with Alzheimer's disease.

☐ **Testamentary trust.** A testamentary trust is a trust that is created upon execution of your loved one's will. Therefore, a testamentary trust *must* be described in your loved one's last will and testament. Because a testamentary trust is part of the will, it is created when the will goes through probate court after your loved one's death. This makes a testamentary trust more public than a living trust.

☐ **Revocable trust.** A revocable trust is a trust that can be modified or dissolved during your loved one's lifetime. For example, real estate named in the trust can be sold and new real estate purchased for the trust, or money in an account named in the trust can be added to or spent. In addition, beneficiaries can be changed in a revocable trust. The designation of revocable trust generally only refers to a living trust (i.e., a *revocable living trust*), because testamentary trusts are always revocable until your loved one's death.

☐ **Irrevocable trust.** An irrevocable trust is a trust that cannot be modified once it is created. Therefore, when your loved one transfers property to an irrevocable trust, they no longer have ownership rights to that property. Living trusts can be irrevocable (i.e., an *irrevocable living trust*), and both living and testamentary trusts become irrevocable upon your loved one's death.

☐ **Purpose-based trusts.** Trusts can be created for a specific purpose, such as managing property or money for a minor child until they reach the age of 18, managing property or money for an adult child with a disability, protecting assets from Medicaid or lawsuits, protecting assets for children from a previous marriage, avoiding certain types of taxes such as an estate tax or gift tax, exempting life insurance payouts from estate taxes, and giving to charitable organizations. Because the types of purpose-based trusts and the tax laws they affect are so diverse, you should speak to a qualified trust agent, lawyer, or financial planner to discuss which trust is right for your loved one.

Checklist: What to put in a trust

- ☐ **Real estate.** Primary residences, vacation homes, rental properties, undeveloped land, corporate buildings, or any other real estate owned by your loved one can be placed in a trust.

- ☐ **Cash.** Cash accounts such as checking accounts, savings accounts, and certificates of deposit can all be placed in a trust.

- ☐ **Investments.** Investments such as stocks, bonds, and mutual funds can be placed in a trust.

- ☐ **Insurance.** Insurance policy payouts can name a trust as the beneficiary. Most commonly, life insurance policies are placed in an irrevocable living trust. Depending on the stipulations in the trust and the type of life insurance policy, this may exempt the policy payout from estate taxes, leaving the beneficiaries with the entire payout rather than only a portion of the payout.

- ☐ **Valuable property.** Other valuable property such as vehicles, jewelry, and other items with monetary or sentimental value can be placed under the ownership of the trust. Remember that *only* property placed in the trust can be managed by the trust.

Checklist: How do I know if my loved one needs a trust?

- ☐ If your loved one has a small estate and no minor or disabled children, a trust is likely not necessary.

- ☐ If your loved one plans to leave their entire estate to their surviving spouse, they likely do not need a trust.

- ☐ If your loved one wants to avoid the costs and time required for probate court, create a trust.

- ☐ If your loved one does not want the contents of their estate to be made public, create a trust.

- ☐ If your loved one has a large estate, especially an estate larger than the current amount that is exempt from estate taxes ($5.43 million in 2015), they should create a trust.

- ☐ If your loved one wants to shelter their estate from Medicaid asset requirements, they will need to form an irrevocable living trust at least five years before they apply for Medicaid assistance.

Checklist: How do I help my loved one create a trust?

- ☐ As with other legal documents, your loved one must be mentally competent to create a trust. Therefore, you should start this process immediately after the diagnosis of Alzheimer's disease if you have not already done so.

- ☐ Identify someone who can help your loved one create a trust document. This may be a lawyer, financial planner, or trust department at a bank.

- ☐ Identify the items your loved one would like to place in the trust. Gather legal paperwork such as deeds, titles, and other proof of ownership.

- ☐ Manually change the owner of every account, property, and any other item to the name of the trust (e.g., instead of the account owner being Joe Smith, the owner should be changed to the Joe Smith Living Trust).

- ☐ Understand that any property not manually transferred to the name of the trust will not be included in the trust.

- ☐ Designate beneficiaries for every item in the trust or otherwise provide instructions for how the property in the trust should be distributed.

- ☐ For revocable trusts, update the document as often as needed. For example, your loved one may need to update the trust document if a new grandchild is born.

☐ Also remember that even if your loved one has a trust, they still need to have a last will and testament for all their possessions that are not named in the trust, such as clothing and household items. Also, guardians of minor children or adult children with disabilities will need to be named in a will rather than a trust.

Once a trust is created, a trustee will be responsible for managing the trust. Choosing a good trustee is vital to having the trust managed honestly and according to your loved one's wishes. The checklists below describe characteristics of a good trustee and responsibilities of a trustee.

Checklist: Characteristics of a good trustee

☐ Meets the state's legal requirements for trustee, including being over the age of 18; however, your loved one will want to choose someone young enough to oversee the trust for many years if needed.

☐ Is a trusted individual, such as the grantor or a spouse, adult child, family lawyer, close friend, bank, or trust company. If you choose a family member, choose wisely so as not to drive a wedge between the trustee and other family members. More than one trustee can be appointed if needed (such as all the adult children of a couple), although doing so is not recommended because it may cause conflicts that cannot be resolved.

☐ Is willing to be trustee.

☐ Has time to manage the trust.

☐ Understands the contents of the trust and how property should be managed.

☐ Understands investing, accounting, and legal responsibilities.

☐ Understands money management principles.

☐ Has integrity, accountability, and good judgment.

☐ Is responsible, organized, and mature.

☐ Is financially secure (to minimize risk of the trustee misusing trust funds for their own purposes).

☐ If choosing a bank or trust company, choose one that has a good reputation, longevity, sufficient capital, and liability insurance.

Checklist: Responsibilities of a trustee

☐ Carefully manage the property in the trust based on your loved one's wishes.

☐ Seek the good of your loved one rather than the good of the beneficiaries.

☐ Weigh the importance of different options to determine which option is closest to your loved one's wishes; be unbiased when making decisions about the trust.

☐ Oversee management of investments, property, and other trust accounts.

☐ Make prudent investments with your loved one's money.

☐ Buy or sell property.

☐ Rent or lease property.

☐ Pay bills as needed from the trust cash accounts.

☐ File and pay income tax for the trust as needed.

☐ Keep records and perform accounting procedures for the trust accounts.

☐ Keep up with changing laws that affect the trust and the responsibilities of the trustee.

☐ Recognize problems and seek the advice of professionals as needed.

☐ Maintain effective communication with your loved one and beneficiaries of the trust.

☐ Disburse money and property to beneficiaries.

☐ Maintain confidentiality about sensitive trust information.

Other Legal Documents and Roles

Although not as common, several other legal documents may be used to help your loved one make healthcare, financial, or other decisions. Some of these documents become either inactive or active based on your loved one's mental competence or death, some are appointed by a physician, and some are drawn up by the court system if your loved one has neglected to make legal documents before their incapacitation. These include documents related to general and springing power of attorney, as well as appointment of a healthcare proxy, conservator, guardian, administrator, representative payee, and/or VA fiduciary. Still other legal documents that may be useful for your loved one to create include a social media will and an ethical will.

Power of Attorney

In addition to the durable power of attorney mentioned earlier in the book, there are two other kinds of power of attorney: the general power of attorney and the springing power of attorney.

General Power of Attorney

The *general power of attorney* (usually just called a "power of attorney") is someone who has been appointed to make financial decisions for another person. Often, a power of attorney is set up for a specific purpose, which is stated in the power of attorney document; once that purpose is fulfilled, the document is no longer valid. For example, if you live in one state but hold property in another state, you may set up a power of attorney authorizing someone in the other state to sell your property for you.

A distinguishing factor of a power of attorney compared to a durable power of attorney is that it is only viable while the grantor is legally competent. Once the grantor has been declared incompetent, the power of attorney document is no longer viable. Therefore, a power of attorney that is not durable is not recommended for individuals with Alzheimer's disease.

Springing Power of Attorney

In contrast to a general power of attorney, a *springing power of attorney* is only effective once an individual is no longer mentally competent. Although this may seem like a good option for someone with Alzheimer's disease, the process of declaring someone legally incompetent can be difficult, because different people may have different ideas about what constitutes competence versus incompetence. During the time it takes to declare your loved one officially incompetent, your loved one must continue making their own financial and healthcare decisions when they shouldn't be. Therefore, using a durable power of attorney is best for individuals with Alzheimer's disease.

Healthcare Proxy

In some states, a healthcare agent is also called a healthcare proxy or medical power of attorney. However, a *healthcare proxy* or *healthcare surrogate* can also refer to someone who is appointed by a physician to make medical decisions for an individual who is medically incapacitated but doesn't have a healthcare agent or a court-appointed guardian. In this regard, the individual has no control over whom the physician chooses to be their healthcare proxy. The physician often chooses a close loved one who is with the individual, such as a spouse or adult child. Once appointed, the healthcare proxy has similar responsibilities as the healthcare. To avoid needing a healthcare proxy, your loved one should sign a durable power of attorney for healthcare while they are still mentally competent.

Conservator and/or Guardian

Another alternative for individuals who do not have a durable power of attorney for healthcare or finances is to have the court appoint a conservator or guardian to make healthcare and financial decisions. In some states, the terms conservator and guardian mean the same thing. However, traditionally a *conservator* is a court-appointed individual who oversees an incapacitated individual's financial matters, and a *guardian* is a court-appointed individual who oversees an incapacitated individual's personal matters, such as healthcare decisions and where to live. The court will state the powers granted to the conservator or guardian. Usually the court will only appoint a conservator or guardian if testing reveals that the individual is legally incompetent.

If your loved one became incompetent before realizing they needed power of attorney documents or simply refused to sign a power of attorney for healthcare or finances, you or your loved one's family members can petition the court for rights of conservatorship or guardianship. The court will first have to determine whether your loved one is mentally incompetent; if so, the court will then appoint someone to be the conservator or guardian. This may or may not be the person who petitioned the court for conservatorship or guardianship. Once this ruling is in place, the appointed person then has the same rights and responsibilities as a durable power of attorney for healthcare and/or a durable power of attorney for finances, depending on the court's ruling. If your loved one doesn't agree with the ruling, they have the right to object to the conservatorship or guardianship. In addition, if there appears to be conflict among family members regarding the choice of guardian or conservator, the court may choose a neutral party rather than a family member.

Although appointing a conservator or guardian is helpful, it should only be used as a last resort if your loved one is incapacitated and does not have durable power of attorney documents in place, because the court proceedings can take as long as one year to complete. In addition, if a conservator or guardian is appointed before a durable power of attorney can be located or identified, the conservator or guardian has legal authority, not the person named in the durable power of attorney.

Guardian of Minor Children

In addition to appointing someone to be guardian for your loved one, the courts may need to appoint a guardian for your loved one's minor children or adult children with disabilities if your loved one becomes unable to care for them. A last will and testament is used to dictate guardianship of minor children after your loved one's death, and a clause can be added that the same individual should care for the children if your loved one becomes incapacitated.

In addition, other legal documents can be used specifically for the purpose of transferring guardianship while your loved one is alive but incapacitated. For this purpose, your loved one will need to create a nomination of guardianship (also called a parental appointment of a guardian) or joint guardianship document. A *nomination of guardianship* document names the person (or people) that your loved one chooses to have guardianship of their children if they become incapacitated. A *joint guardianship* document allows your loved one to transfer legal rights to another individual while they are still alive and keep to also parental rights until their death; this is the recommended legal document for individuals with Alzheimer's disease.

Accepting guardianship of minor children or an adult with a disability is a major responsibility. Therefore, choosing an appropriate guardian is of utmost importance. In general, it is best to appoint the same guardian in a guardianship document as is listed in the last will and testament in order to ease the transition for the child. In addition, if guardianship will go to a couple, both the husband and wife should be listed in the guardianship document. An alternative guardian should also be listed in case the primary guardian is unavailable.

Once the guardian has begun their duties, they will need to care for that child as if the child is their own. This includes taking on the financial responsibilities that come with raising a child unless the child's parent has made financial provisions for their care through a will or trust. The checklist below indicates things to consider when choosing a good guardian for children.

Checklist: Things to consider when choosing a good guardian for children

- ☐ Does the individual meet the legal requirements for a guardian, including being over the age of 18?

- ☐ Is the individual willing to accept guardianship of all of your loved one's children? Or would the children be placed in different homes?

- ☐ Does your loved one's child prefer one particular individual to be their guardian if their parents become incapacitated?

- ☐ Does the individual have a genuine interest in the well-being and care of your loved one's children?

- ☐ Is the individual physically, emotionally, and financially able to care for your loved one's children?

- ☐ Is the individual willing to spend their own money to care for your loved one's children?

- ☐ Does the individual get along well with your loved one's children?

- ☐ Will the individual provide a stable home and family life for your loved one's children?

- ☐ Does the individual share the morals, values, and beliefs that your loved one has tried to instill in their children?

- ☐ Will the individual discipline your loved one's children in the same manner your loved one would discipline them?

- ☐ Is the individual willing to accept full responsibility for the children's actions, even if they get in trouble with the law?

- ☐ If living with this individual, would your loved one's children be able to attend the same school they did previously? Or would they have to change school systems?

- ☐ If the child (or adult) has a disability, does the individual have the time, energy, and skill needed to care for a person with a disability?

Administrator

If your loved one dies without a last will and testament, the courts will appoint an administrator to oversee the distribution of your loved one's estate. The administrator may or may not be someone your loved one would have chosen. In most states, the court will name your loved one's spouse as the administrator. If your loved one has no spouse, the next of kin is usually selected. In general, the administrator has the same responsibilities as a named executor. However, an executor may have additional duties compared to an administrator based on the stipulations of the will (such as stipulations involving the sale of real estate). The administrator will also have to post bond for the estate, which is a cost determined by probate court. This cost is often waived if your loved one has a will and a named executor.

Representative Payee and/or VA Fiduciary

An individual acting as the attorney-in-fact for finances does not have the legal right to manage income from Social Security or veterans benefits. If your loved one is eligible to receive benefits from these sources, the government names the agents who will manage these benefits. A representative payee is named to manage Social Security benefits, and a VA fiduciary is named to manage veterans benefits. The government may appoint the same individual or entity as the durable power of attorney for finances, but they may also choose someone else instead.

Social Media Will

As we move further into the digital age, more individuals are opening social media accounts, including accounts on Facebook, Twitter, LinkedIn, Google, and others. Privacy laws prevent anyone other than the original owner from accessing these accounts. Thus, if your loved one has any social media accounts, they should consider writing a social media will. First, your loved one should consult the privacy policies for each social media site. Then, in the will, your loved one should write how they would like the account handled after their incapacitation or death based on the privacy policies of the site. Some sites may allow a page to remain open as a memorial, or they may require that your loved one's page be closed or canceled. Your loved one should provide the executor of their social media will with a list of accounts, login IDs, and passwords. The executor should also obtain a copy of your loved one's death certificate, as some companies require this in order for someone else to make changes to the account.

Ethical Will

Although an ethical will is not technically a legal document, it can be used to pass on values, memories, and beliefs to those left behind just as much as a last will and testament can be used to pass on physical possessions. An ethical will is usually a letter or video that provides a last message to close family members and friends about the things that hold most value for your loved one. It can include statements of personal or religious beliefs, hopes and dreams for children or grandchildren, words of encouragement, lessons your loved one has learned in life, or forgiveness or apologies for past hurts. A loved one who is young with small children may want to write letters for children to open on important dates such as birthdays, graduations, weddings, etc. Ethical wills can also be used to try to mend broken relationships. For individuals with Alzheimer's disease who will slowly lose their mental capabilities, writing an ethical will is a great way to preserve memories and solidify relationships before your loved one is no longer able to communicate.

Dealing with Conflict

Caring for a loved one with Alzheimer's disease brings with it many decisions, complications, and stresses. For many families, daily decisions about healthcare, finances, and other responsibilities are a heavy burden that often brings out the worst in everyone. These problems are magnified in blended or dysfunctional families. Dealing with family conflict adds more stress to an already stressful situation, especially for family members who are involved in caring for your loved one in a legal capacity. My friend Amy and I are both only children, so we did not have any disputes with family members. However, there are a million stories of families being torn apart because of decisions made by one sibling or parent that the other family members did not agree with. The checklists below note common causes of disagreements and provide ways to resolve or prevent conflicts.

Checklist: Common causes of conflict

☐ Family members have different opinions about the best choices for medical care, especially at the end of life. This is especially common between a spouse and adult children.

☐ Family members disagree about what they think your loved one would want in any particular situation, including both healthcare and financial decisions.

☐ Family members disagree about who should be the primary caregiver for your loved one, or one family member refuses to participate in caregiving responsibilities.

☐ A family member is not carrying an equal burden of caring for your loved one or feels like they are carrying the whole burden of caring for your loved one.

☐ A family member is resented for living far away and not contributing to your loved one's care.

☐ Family members disagree on who should provide housing for your loved one if your loved one can no longer live alone.

☐ Family members disagree on who should be your loved one's physician or which long-term care facility they should move into.

☐ Children from blended families disagree on how your loved one should be cared for.

☐ Children from a first marriage resent the involvement of a spouse or children from a second marriage.

☐ Family members allow childhood conflicts or rivalries to infiltrate the decision-making process concerning your loved one's care.

- ☐ Family members disagree about or don't fully understand your loved one's physical and mental limitations.

- ☐ Family members have different opinions about the distribution of assets, especially for expensive items or items with great sentimental value.

- ☐ A family member insists that they want their inheritance now before your loved one's death.

- ☐ A family member wants to "borrow" money from your loved one's estate.

- ☐ Family members disagree about how to pay for your loved one's care.

- ☐ Family members disagree about the contents of a legal document.

- ☐ Family members disagree about how to deal with the scams your loved one has fallen prey to.

- ☐ Family members feel anger, frustration, resentment, fear, helplessness, or grief over your loved one's condition.

- ☐ A family member is in denial about your loved one's condition, or your loved one is in denial about their own condition or diagnosis.

Checklist: Strategies to prevent or resolve conflict

- ☐ Listen carefully to family members' opinions, and respect their opinions. Keep an open mind and try to understand their point of view.

- ☐ Keep lines of communication open between family members. Try not to exclude any family members from this discussion, even if they live far away or are known for their poor choices and irresponsibility.

- ☐ Keep family members informed about your loved one's condition as it changes.

- ☐ Schedule regular face-to-face meetings for the family to discuss changes in your loved one's situation. Use these meeting as a forum for anyone to voice feelings of experiencing caregiver burnout.

☐ Talk honestly about your feelings and burdens with other family members or friends. Sometimes sharing the burden can help lighten the load for everyone.

☐ If you are the legal representative, understand your legal rights when making decisions about your loved one's healthcare and/or finances while also allowing other family members to share their opinions and provide insight when making big decisions, such as when to move your loved one from their home.

☐ Express appreciation for the care that is being provided by others.

☐ Make a list of caregiving tasks, including how much time, money, and effort is needed to complete the task. Divide tasks as evenly as possible among family members based on skills and availability. Tasks may include cooking, cleaning, providing hygiene care, doing grocery shopping, performing home maintenance, paying bills, driving to appointments, and many others.

☐ Plan for anticipated changes in your loved one's needs as the disease progresses.

☐ Avoid physically or verbally attacking others who have a different opinion than you do.

☐ Try not to blame others for bad situations; don't criticize others for not participating in your loved one's care or not performing care "correctly."

☐ Resolve childhood conflicts between family members to allow everyone to participate in decisions and caregiving without letting past issues disrupt the current situation.

☐ Seek help from a neutral third party when disagreements occur. For healthcare disagreements, consult your loved one's physician or other medical professional. For financial disagreements, consult your loved one's attorney or trustee (if the trustee is not a family member). For other disagreements, consult a counselor, pastor, mediator, social worker, or shared friend. Websites that list mediators by state are provided in the Resources section at the end of the book.

☐ Encourage family members to join a support group for families of individuals with Alzheimer's disease.

☐ Hire help to provide caregiving services or take care of household tasks.

☐ If you live far away, offer to help in any way you can. Offer to provide emotional support to caregivers through phone calls, letters, or cards. Offer financial support if needed. Visit as your schedule allows.

☐ Make sure all family members and caregivers are taking care of themselves by getting regular sleep, nutritious meals, and adequate exercise.

Conclusion

The creation of legal documents is a detailed matter that should not be taken lightly. The selection of a healthcare agent, attorney-in-fact, executor, or trustee requires careful consideration, and the named representative will have heavy responsibility placed on them after committing to the job. In addition, determining healthcare choices for the end of life and determining how property will be distributed will require critical thinking and thorough planning. If your loved one has been diagnosed with Alzheimer's disease, many of these decisions will become too hard for them once the disease progresses. Therefore, creating legal documents as soon as possible after diagnosis is essential. Both you and your loved one will feel a weight lifted off your shoulders once major decisions about the future have been made and these legal documents are in place.

ABOUT THE AUTHORS

Laura Town

Laura Town has authored numerous publications of special interest to the aging population. She has expertise in the field of finance as a co-author on *Finance: Foundations of Financial Institutions and Management*, published by John Wiley and Sons, and she has contributed to several online nursing courses and texts. She has also written for the American Medical Writers Association, and her work has been published by the American Society of Journalists and Authors. As an editor, Laura has worked with Pearson Education, Prentice Hall, McGraw-Hill Higher Education, John Wiley and Sons, and the University of Pennsylvania to create both on-ground and online courses and texts. She is currently the President-Elect of the Indiana chapter of the American Medical Writers Association.

Karen Kassel

Karen Kassel received her Ph.D. in pharmacology from the Department of Pharmacology and Experimental Neurosciences at the University of Nebraska Medical Center in Omaha, where she was the recipient of an American Heart Association fellowship and several regional and national awards for her research on G protein-coupled receptor signaling in airways. She then pursued post-doctoral research projects at the University of North Carolina–Chapel Hill and the University of Kansas Medical Center, again receiving fellowships from the PhRMA Foundation and the American Heart Association, respectively. She has published research in the *American Journal of Pathology*, *Journal of Biological Chemistry*, and *Journal of Pharmacology and Experimental Therapeutics*. In 2012, Karen joined the editorial staff at WilliamsTown Communications, an editing firm that specializes in educational products for undergraduate- and graduate-level students. At WTC, Karen specializes in producing educational products related to the sciences and healthcare. In addition, Karen is board-certified for editing life sciences (BELS-certified).

A NOTE FROM THE AUTHORS

Thank you for purchasing our book! Worldwide, over 40 million people suffer from Alzheimer's disease, and that number is expected to increase significantly within the next 15 years. In the United States, five million people have the disease, and that is expected to triple by the year 2050.

Despite these large numbers, you may feel alone. I (Laura) know that when I started caring for my father, who had early-onset Alzheimer's disease, I felt alone. Although my father has passed away, I am haunted by what he suffered and how difficult it was to care for him. However, now I know that there are people, resources, and organizations that can help others going through this same struggle.

We recognize that caregivers have emotional, physical, and financial challenges. We hope that the information in the *Alzheimer's Roadmap* series will ease some of your stress. The legal documents discussed in this book will help you prepare for that inevitable day when your loved one is no longer able to make their own decisions about healthcare and finances. In addition, we have included resources at the end of each book to provide additional information to help you through this process.

If you have any questions for us, feel free to post them on Laura Town's Amazon Author Central page or reach out to either author via Twitter: @laurawtown and @KarenKassel1. We would appreciate it if you would take the time to review our book on Amazon, as our book's visibility on Amazon depends on reviews.

More Titles from Laura Town and Karen Kassel

Alzheimer's Roadmap series:

- ☐ *Long-Term Care Insurance, Power of Attorney, Wealth Management, and Other First Steps*

- ☐ *Dementia, Alzheimer's Disease Stages, Treatment Options, and Other Medical Considerations*

- ☐ *Home Safety Checklist Guide and Caregiver Resources for Medication Safety, Driving, and Wandering*

- ☐ *Home Care, Long-Term Care, Memory Care Units, and Other Living Arrangements*

- ☐ *Caregiver Resources for Helping with Activities of Daily Living*

- ☐ *Nutrition for Brain Health: Fighting Dementia*

- ☐ *Caregiver Resources: From Independence to a Memory Care Unit*

   (This book combines information from *Home Safety Checklist Guide and Caregiver Resources for Medication Safety, Driving, and Wandering* and information from *Home Care, Long-Term Care, Memory Care Units, and Other Living Arrangements.*)

RESOURCES

Information about Alzheimer's Disease

Alzheimer's Association
225 N. Michigan Avenue, Floor 17
Chicago, IL 60601-7633
Phone: 800-272-3900
Fax: 866-699-1246
Email: info@alz.org
Website: http://www.alz.org

Alzheimer's Disease Education and Referral (ADEAR) Center
P.O. Box 8250
Silver Spring, MD 20907-8250
Phone: 800-438-4380
Website: www.nia.nih.gov/alzheimers

Alzheimer's Foundation of America
322 Eighth Avenue, 7th Floor
New York, NY 10001
Phone: 866-232-8484
Fax: 646-638-1546
Website: www.alzfdn.org

Information about Legal Advice or Lawyers

Administration on Aging Eldercare Locator
Phone: 800-677-1116
Website: http://eldercare.gov/eldercare.NET/Public/index.aspx
*Find connections for legal assistance and many other topics

American Bar Association
321 N. Clark Street
Chicago, IL 60654
Phone: 800-285-2221
Website: www.americanbar.org
*Provides legal information related to many topics

National Academy of Elder Law Attorneys
1577 Spring Hill Road, Suite 220
Vienna, VA 22182
Phone: 703-942-5711
Website: http://www.naela.org/Public
*Lists all certified elder law attorneys in the United States

National Institute on Aging
Building 31, Room 5C27
31 Center Drive, MSC 2292
Bethesda, MD 20892
Phone: 800-222-2225
Email: niaic@nia.nih.gov
Website: http://www.nia.nih.gov/
Specific helpful website:
http://www.nia.nih.gov/alzheimers/legal-and-financial-issues-people-alzheimers-disease-resource-list
*Provides a list of resources for legal and financial issues

National Legal Resource Center
Website: www.nlrc.aoa.gov
*Provides information about legal issues and legal resources

National Senior Citizens Law Center
1444 Eye Street NW, Suite 1100
Washington, DC 20005
Phone: 202-289-6976
Website: www.nsclc.org
*Provides limited free legal information

Information about Organ Donation and Other Advance Directives

Donate Life America
701 East Byrd Street, 16th floor
Richmond, VA 23219
Phone: 804-377-3580
Website: www.donatelife.net

Health Resources and Services Administration
Phone: 888-275-4772
Website: www.organdonor.gov

POLST (Physician Orders for Life-Sustaining Treatment)
Website: www.polst.org
Specific helpful website:
http://capolst.org/wp-content/uploads/2014/01/CAPOLSTform2011.pdf
*Provides an example POLST form

Put It In Writing
American Hospital Association
155 North Wacker Drive
Chicago, IL 60606
Phone: 800-424-4301
Website: www.putitinwriting.org

The Living Bank
P.O. Box 6725
Houston, TX 77265
Phone: 800-528-2971
Website: www.livingbank.org

Information about Resolving Family Conflict

Alzheimer's Association
Website: http://www.alz.org/apps/we_can_help/support_groups.asp
*Search for local support groups

Elder Decisions
30 Walpole Street
Norwood, MA 02062
Phone: 866-736-9008
Email: info@elderdecisions.com
Website: www.elderdecisions.com
*Mediators will travel to your location

Mediate.com
Website: http://www.mediate.com/index.cfm
*Provides links for finding mediators by state/city and country

Mediation.org
Website: http://www.mediation.org/
*Search for mediators by state, city, and/or zip code

Other

AARP
601 E Street, NW
Washington, DC 20049
Phone: 888-OUR-AARP (888-687-2277)
Email: member@aarp.org
Website: http://www.aarp.org/
*Information for individuals over age 50

National Council on Aging Benefits CheckUp
1901 L Street NW, 4th Floor
Washington, DC 20036
Phone: 202-479-1200
Website: https://www.benefitscheckup.org/
*Helps find government benefits for which your loved one qualifies

National Hospice and Palliative Care Organization
1731 King Street
Alexandria, VA 22314
Phone: 800-658-8898
Website: www.caringinfo.org
*Provides information about hospice services

Alzheimer's Roadmap series
Purchase from Amazon.com, CreateSpace.com, and on Kindle and other devices:

- *Long-Term Care Insurance, Power of Attorney, Wealth Management, and Other First Steps*
- *Dementia, Alzheimer's Disease Stages, Treatment Options, and Other Medical Considerations*
- *Home Safety Checklist Guide and Caregiver Resources for Medication Safety, Driving, and Wandering*
- *Home Care, Long-Term Care, Memory Care Units, and Other Living Arrangements*
- *Caregiver Resources for Helping with Activities of Daily Living*
- *Nutrition for Brain Health: Fighting Dementia*
- *Caregiver Resources: From Independence to a Memory Care Unit*

    (This book combines information from *Home Safety Checklist Guide and Caregiver Resources for Medication Safety, Driving, and Wandering* and information from *Home Care, Long-Term Care, Memory Care Units, and Other Living Arrangements*.)

REFERENCE LIST

Alzheimer's Association. (2014). Retrieved from http://www.alz.org/

American Bar Association. (2014). Retrieved from http://www.americanbar.org/
aba.html

American Health Lawyers Association. (2014). A guide to legal issues in life-limiting
conditions. Retrieved from http://www.healthlawyers.org/hlresources/PI/
InfoSeries/Documents/LLC%202nd%20Edition.pdf

Bryant, K. (n.d.). 37 types of trusts used to protect assets from creditors, the
government, and other predators. Retrieved from http://www.eldercarelaw
jacksonville.com/2012/04/25/types-of-trusts-protect-assets

Burroughs, A. (2011). When your client has Alzheimer's. Retrieved from
http://wealthmanagement.com/financial-planning/when-your-client-has-
alzheimer-s

California POLST form. (2011). Retrieved from http://capolst.org/wp-content/
uploads/2014/01/CAPOLSTform2011.pdf

Candito, J. (2011). Executor or administrator? What's the difference? Retrieved
from http://blueashattorney.com/2011/10/executor-or-administrator-whats-
the-difference/

CaregiverStress.com. (2014). Retrieved from http://www.caregiverstress.com/

Casey, J. (2008). How to hire an elder law attorney. Retrieved from
http://alzheimers.about.com/lw/Health-Medicine/Geriatric-Health/How-to-
Hire-an-Eldercare-Attorney.htm

Celebrations of Life. (n.d.). Ethical wills/Legacy letters. Retrieved from
http://celebrationsoflife.net/ethicalwills/

Consumer Financial Protection Bureau. (2013). Managing someone else's money:
Help for agents under a power of attorney. Retrieved from http://files.
consumerfinance.gov/f/201310_cfpb_lay_fiduciary_guides_agents.pdf

Dimick, C. (2011). Sorting out advance directives. *Journal of AHIMA, 82*(1): 26–30.

Family Caregiver Alliance. (2003). Caregiving and sibling relationships: Challenges
and opportunities. Retrieved from https://caregiver.org/caregiving-and-sibling-
relationships-challenges-and-opportunities

FindLaw. (n.d.). How to establish guardianship of a child FAQs. Retrieved from
http://family.findlaw.com/guardianship/how-to-establish-guardianship-of-a-
child-faqs.html

Fisher Center for Alzheimer's Research Foundation. (2014). Retrieved from
http://www.alzinfo.org/

The Florida Bar. (2014). Do you have a will? Retrieved from
https://www.floridabar.org/tfb/TFBConsum.nsf/48e76203493b82ad85256709
0070c9b9/a0091ab18d4875d085256b2f006c5b75?OpenDocument

The Free Dictionary. (n.d.) Executors and administrators. Retrieved from
http://legal-dictionary.thefreedictionary.com/Executors+and+Administrators

Just Health and Family Law. (2010). Guardianship agreements. Retrieved from
http://www.justhealthandfamily.com/guardianship-agreements.html

Leonard, W. (2014). Alzheimer's disease complications. Retrieved from
http://www.healthline.com/health/alzheimers-disease-complications#
Overview1

Life Issues Institute. (n.d.). Planning for future medical decisions: How to prepare a
personalized living will. Retrieved from http://www.lifeissues.org/euthanasia/
pdf/your_life_your_choices.pdf

Living Trust Network. (2014). Retrieved from http://livingtrustnetwork.com/

Matthiessen, C. (n.d.). Caring for elderly relatives: How to handle family conflicts.
Retrieved from http://www.caring.com/articles/family-conflict

Mayo Clinic. (2012). Alzheimer's: Dealing with family conflict. Retrieved from
http://www.mayoclinic.org/healthy-living/caregivers/in-depth/alzheimers/art-
20047365

National Hospice and Palliative Care Organization. (n.d.). Retrieved from
http://www.caringinfo.org/i4a/pages/index.cfm?pageid=1

National Institute on Aging. (n.d.). Retrieved from http://www.nia.nih.gov

New York Organ Donor Network. (2014). What organs can be donated? Retrieved
from http://www.donatelifeny.org/about-donation/what-can-be-donated/

Pareto, C. (n.d.). Estate planning: Introduction to trusts. Retrieved from
http://www.investopedia.com/university/estate-planning/estate-planning6.asp

RBC Wealth Management. (2014). Transferring wealth: Creating a legacy through estate planning. Retrieved from http://www.rbcwm-usa.com/resources/file-687698.pdf

U.S. Government. (2014). Writing a will. Retrieved from http://www.usa.gov/topics/money/personal-finance/wills.shtml

VA Estate Planner. (2012). The trustee. Retrieved from http://vaestateplanner.wordpress.com/

CPSIA information can be obtained
at www.ICGtesting.com
Printed in the USA
LVOW03s2018120117
520749LV00006B/549/P

FEB 2 7 2017

9 781943 414000